D0408230

Made up

Laura Jenkinson

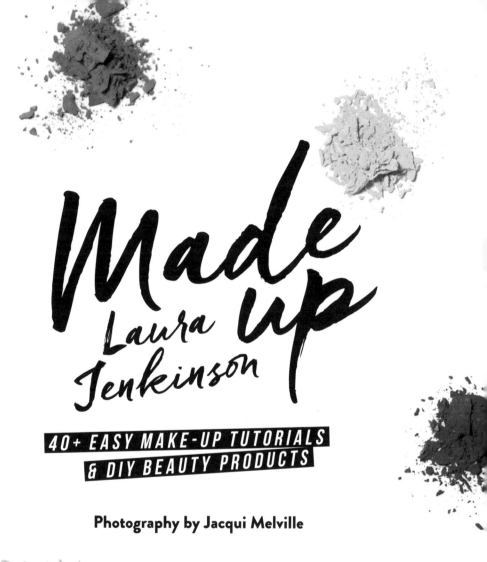

Made Up

Laura Jenkinson

40+ EASY MAKE-UP TUTORIALS & DIY BEAUTY PRODUCTS

Photography by Jacqui Melville

hardie grant books

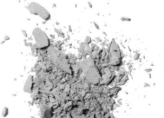

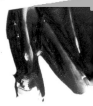

CONT

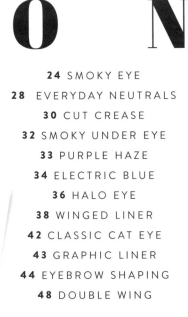

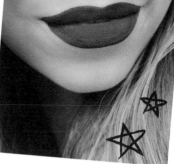

E N T S

HELLO

Make-up can be used to totally transform yourself or subtly enhance your best features. I love working as a make-up artist – I've had the chance to work at London Fashion Week, on music videos and even at murder mystery parties! It's so rewarding to help my clients achieve their perfect look, whether it's soft and pretty or bold and fierce.

Since growing a following on Instagram (@laurajenkinson) by posting my unique looks, creating characters and illusions by drawing on my face and focusing on my mouth and teeth, I've been featured in Reddit, Buzzfeed and *Cosmopolitan*. Make-up has brought me freedom, excitement and fantastic opportunities.

Made Up is something I have only ever dreamt of creating, and I can't wait to share it all with you. I have carefully selected my favourite products, techniques, tips and how-tos, and answered the most commonly asked questions from friends, family and clients. From step-by-steps on contouring, highlighting and applying false eyelashes to full face looks perfect for festivals and date nights, this book will show you how to use make-up to its full potential.

You'll learn to apply eye make-up ranging from everyday neutrals to dramatic graphic liner, and find out how to choose the best lipstick and blusher shades for your skin tone. I hope to inspire you to create new and eye-catching makeovers that will fill you with confidence and help you look and feel incredible!

Laura Jenkinson

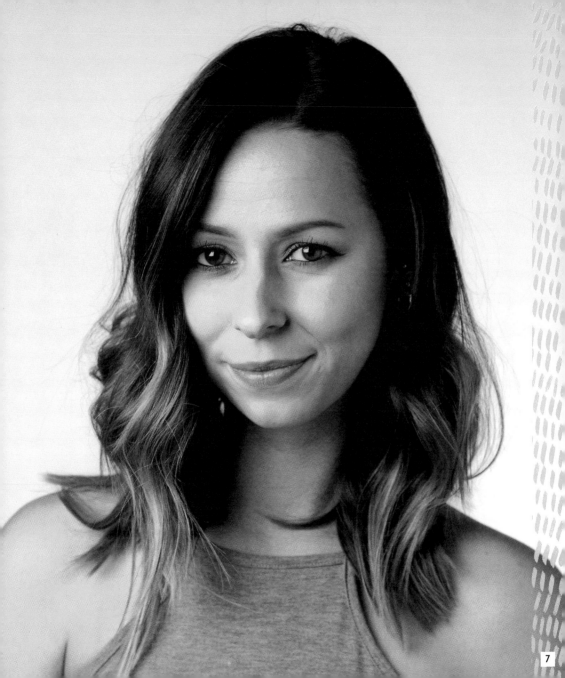

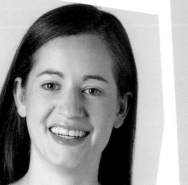
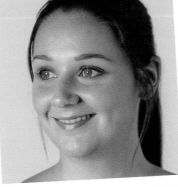
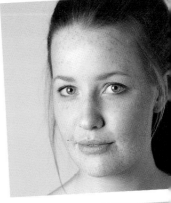

Skincare
ROUTINE

Studies have found that almost 2 kg (5 lb) of chemicals from make-up and beauty products is absorbed into our skin each year, so it's important to know what we are applying to our faces and to take extra care in doing so. Our skin is our largest organ, so we have to look after it, and the best way to do this is to perfect our skincare routine.

We've all heard that we should cleanse, tone and moisturise. Here's a breakdown of what each term means and the importance of each process:

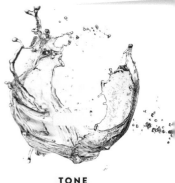

CLEANSE

A gentle facial cleanser will remove make-up, oils, dirt and anything else your skin has picked up throughout the day. Apply all over your face and leave to absorb for half a minute or so, then remove with cotton wool pads or warm water.

TONE

A toner softens, smooths and (you guessed it) tones the skin. Most toners have skin-repairing ingredients, which help to replenish the skin. They also remove any trace of cleanser that might still be on your skin.

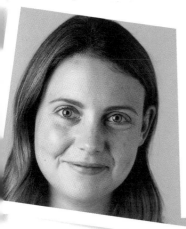
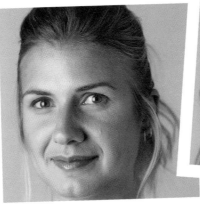
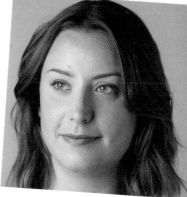

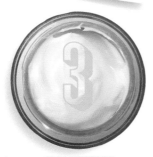

MOISTURISE

(The best part!) Moisturisers contain ingredients that help skin look healthier and younger. As we get older our skin begins to change, as it gradually starts to lose its natural moisturising properties. Using a daily moisturiser helps to keep our skin feeling fresh, young and rejuvenated. When applied in the morning, it also helps make-up stay on longer throughout the day.

Now we have established why these steps are important, it's equally essential to make sure you're using the right products.

To make your skincare routine effective and achieve the best results, you need to select products that are tailored to your skin type. Just because your friend raves about one product, it doesn't mean that will necessarily work for you and your skin type.

The best and most inexpensive way to do this is first to determine your skin type (see pages 10-11). Then go to any beauty/skincare shop or counter and ask for a variety of testers suited to that skin type. Try them out and identify which works best for you and gives the best results.

You've probably heard it a hundred times, but a good night's sleep and **DRINKING LOTS OF WATER** *really does do wonders for your skin!*

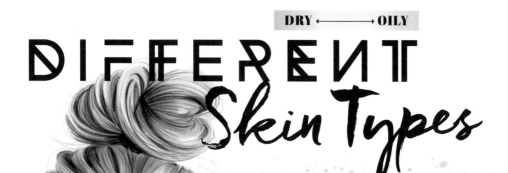

DIFFERENT *Skin Types*

OILY
All-over shine; large pores; frequent blemishes. Fewer lines and wrinkles.

NORMAL
Even complexion; small pores; few breakouts.

DRY

Small pores; face feels tight. Cheeks and/or chin can become flaky and dry.

COMBINATION

Oily T-zone; cheeks are normal to dry. Breakouts on chin, nose, cheeks and forehead.

SENSITIVE

Blotchy, dry/red patches; rosacea, delicate/thin skin. Sensitive to products.

Brushes from my collection

Using the correct tools is essential to creating that perfect finish. Here I have carefully selected a range of essential brushes for your make-up kit. Whether you're a pro or simply a make-up lover, my cruelty-free, chic collection is a must-have for your make-up bag.

1
ANGLED EYELINER BRUSH (106)
This brush gives you perfect precision to create winged liner. It can also be used to fill in eyebrows with a gel or powder product.

2
EYEBROW COMB (117)
Otherwise known as a spoolie, this brush is perfect for brushing your eyebrow hairs into the same direction before you begin filling them in. It also blends out product if you happen to apply too much, creating a more natural finish.

3
LIP BRUSH (118)
This brush gives you complete precision when applying lipstick, leaving sharp, clean edges.

4
EYESHADOW BRUSH (128)
This small, flat brush is perfect for applying eyeshadow all over the lid. I also use it as a concealer brush.

5
BLENDING BRUSH (136)
This small, soft brush is used for blending out eyeshadow. The brush is designed to do most the work for you; if you hold it gently and sweep it back and forth, it will diffuse the make-up into the skin, leaving no harsh lines.

6
FAN BRUSH (170)
This is the perfect brush for applying a light dusting of highlighter on the cheekbones. It also works to sweep away any product that may have dropped down under the eyes after applying eyeshadow.

Brushes can be purchased from
WWW.LAURA-JENKINSON.COM

7
FLAT FOUNDATION BRUSH (180)

This brush is typically used for applying liquid foundation and is probably the quickest and easiest way to do so. I also use this brush to apply primer, rather then using my fingers.

8
BUFFING BRUSH (184)

This brush is used to apply liquid or cream foundation in circular motions for heavier coverage and a flawless finish.

9
STIPPLE BRUSH (187)

This has finer fibres near the top of the brush. These fibres create light coverage with liquid or cream foundation and can also be used to create that finished airbrushed look.

10
ANGLED POWDER BRUSH (197)

The ideal brush for contouring – because of the angle and size, this brush does most of the work for you.

11
POWDER BRUSH (196)

This soft brush picks up loose powder to apply on your T-zone, under your eyes and around the nose and mouth area to stop foundation from creasing. It is also perfect for a touch of blush on the apples of the cheeks.

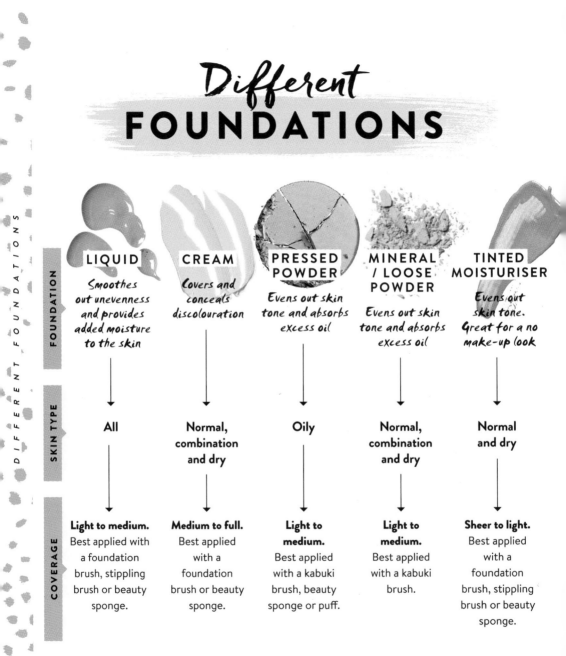

Different
FOUNDATIONS

FOUNDATION	LIQUID	CREAM	PRESSED POWDER	MINERAL / LOOSE POWDER	TINTED MOISTURISER
	Smoothes out unevenness and provides added moisture to the skin	Covers and conceals discolouration	Evens out skin tone and absorbs excess oil	Evens out skin tone and absorbs excess oil	Evens out skin tone. Great for a no make-up look
SKIN TYPE	All	Normal, combination and dry	Oily	Normal, combination and dry	Normal and dry
COVERAGE	**Light to medium.** Best applied with a foundation brush, stippling brush or beauty sponge.	**Medium to full.** Best applied with a foundation brush or beauty sponge.	**Light to medium.** Best applied with a kabuki brush, beauty sponge or puff.	**Light to medium.** Best applied with a kabuki brush.	**Sheer to light.** Best applied with a foundation brush, stippling brush or beauty sponge.

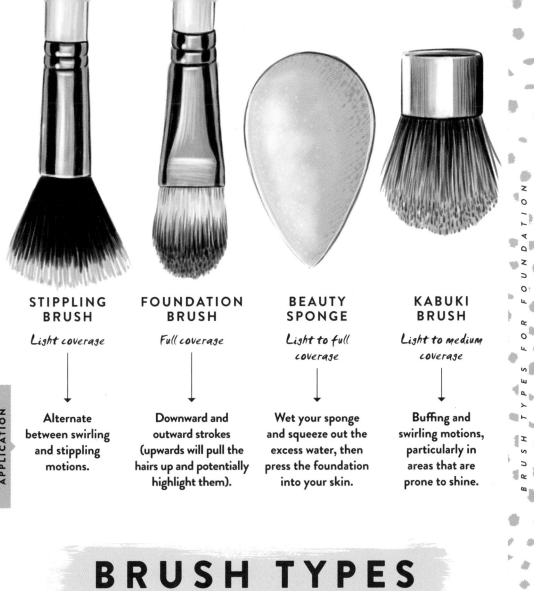

STIPPLING BRUSH

Light coverage

↓

Alternate between swirling and stippling motions.

FOUNDATION BRUSH

Full coverage

↓

Downward and outward strokes (upwards will pull the hairs up and potentially highlight them).

BEAUTY SPONGE

Light to full coverage

↓

Wet your sponge and squeeze out the excess water, then press the foundation into your skin.

KABUKI BRUSH

Light to medium coverage

↓

Buffing and swirling motions, particularly in areas that are prone to shine.

APPLICATION

BRUSH TYPES
for Foundation

Cleaning Your Brushes + Tools

It's not the most exciting task in the world, but it is vital to regularly clean your make-up brushes and tools. Ideally, all brushes and tools should be cleaned after every use but this isn't always possible, especially if you apply make-up every day. However, if you're prone to breakouts or have sensitive skin, you should definitely wash your brushes regularly! Otherwise, aim to clean them at least every two weeks.

BRUSHES

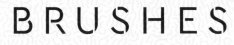

Start off by rinsing the bristles with warm water. Hold the brush downwards to avoid any water getting into the ferrule or handle of the brush, which can weaken the glue. Add a small amount of mild soap, lather up, then rinse with warm water.

If you wish, you can use an alcohol-based industrial cleaner. I see the best results with IPA (isopropyl alcohol, 99.9%). It can be bought online and I recommend it if you are a professional make-up artist, but you must be careful to avoid it getting in your eyes or mouth. IPA thoroughly cleans and disinfects your make-up brushes, more so then a baby shampoo or mild soap will do, killing any bacteria that may be left on the bristles. You also only need a very small amount per brush. If you use IPA, thoroughly rinse it off, remembering to hold the brush downwards with the water and only stopping once the water runs clear.

Most cosmetic brands have their own brush cleaners, which usually contain alcohol, and these are great to use too.

Finally, leave your brushes to dry overnight – in the morning you'll be left with lovely, bacteria-free brushes!

Sponges + Beauty Blenders

Sponges and beauty blenders should be rinsed after every use to keep them in the best condition and to keep germs away. When it's time for a deep clean, rinse the sponge or beauty blender under warm water, then lather a small amount of mild soap (my favourite is Fairy Liquid) into the sponge or beauty blender using your fingers. Rinse thoroughly until the water runs clear. Leave to dry, or alternatively, squeeze out the water and use straight away, as they are great to use when they are slightly damp.

Remember that sponges and beauty blenders don't have as long lifespans as brushes, so you should replace them around every four months.

METAL TOOLS

(TWEEZERS, EYELASH CURLERS ETC)

Sanitise these with an alcohol (IPA)-soaked tissue or cotton pad. Then rinse with water and some antibacterial soap and leave to dry. You should do this after every use to decrease the chance of any skin infections.

Applying FOUNDATION

As a make-up artist, 'How should I apply my foundation?' is definitely one of the most common questions I get asked by friends, family and clients, and it is actually one of the hardest to answer. Every single one of us is so different. We all have different skin types, whether dry, oily or combination, so what works for one person might not work for another. Plus, our skin is constantly changing, so if you haven't found that perfect liquid foundation yet, try mixing it up a bit; you might find you are better suited to a powder foundation.

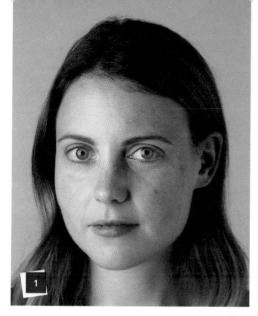

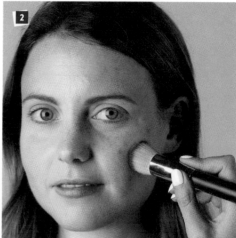

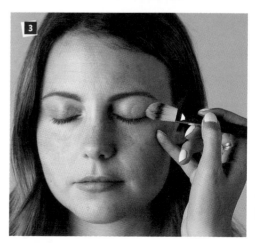

There are different brushes and tools you can use to apply foundation. Some brushes will give you more coverage then others. An explanation of the different brush types can be found on page 15.

1 / The key to getting that flawless look with your skin is to prep it beforehand. Always start with hydrated skin. Cleanse, tone and moisturise (see pages 8–9). Wait 5 minutes after prep to let the products really soak in.

2 / Taking a liquid foundation and a foundation brush, start applying your foundation to the skin in downward and outward strokes.

3 / Don't forget to apply on the eye area too, particularly the eyelids. The colour of our eyelids can sometimes make us appear tired, so making sure your skin tone is even all over will instantly brighten your face and widen your eyes.

APPLYING FOUNDATION

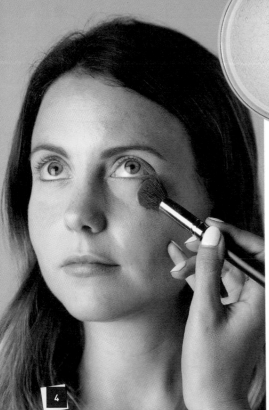

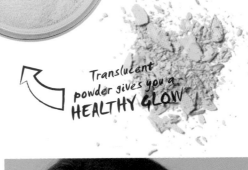

Translucent powder gives you a HEALTHY GLOW

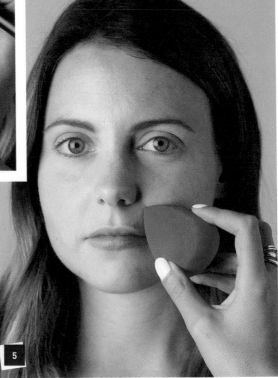

4 / Apply concealer where necessary, such as on spots or dark circles under the eyes. I believe that most coverage can be achieved with foundation and the right tools, so concealer may not always be necessary.

5 / Blend the concealer using a beauty sponge.

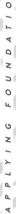

6

6 / Finally, set the foundation with a luminous, translucent powder. This reflects the light and will make your skin glow.

5/10/15 MINUTE MAKE-UP

MAC in EMBARK

No-one has the time or energy to set an hour aside every single morning to do their make-up before the day ahead. Depending on how much time you have, you can start off with a few basic products and gradually build up and add steps. Anything that saves a little time and leaves you with a few extra minutes in bed is worth a try!

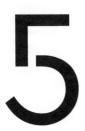

5

1 / MAC Face and Body Foundation gives very sheer and light coverage, but can be built up if required. It also blends easily with fingertips and leaves a fresh and dewy finish.

2 / Japonesque Velvet Touch Blush. Adding a small amount of blush can instantly make you look more awake and fresh (a good trick if you're feeling a little hungover).

3 / Maybelline Great Lash Mascara.

4 / Elizabeth Arden Eight Hour Cream. Perfect moisturiser for the lips and a make-up bag must-have.

1 / Chanel Perfection Lumière foundation set with **Laura Mercier Translucent Loose Setting Powder**. This foundation gives such even coverage and leaves skin looking unblemished and glowing. (Also smells great!)

2 / Kevyn Aucoin bronzer in **Tropical Days** with a touch of **Japonesque Velvet Touch Blush.**

3 / MAC eyeshadow in **Embark** blended out on lash lines.

4 / Maybelline Great Lash Mascara.

5 / Elizabeth Arden Eight Hour Cream.

Anastasia Beverly Hills Liquid Lipstick in DUSTY ROSE

1 / Chanel Perfection Lumière foundation set with **Laura Mercier Translucent Loose Setting Powder.**

2 / Kevyn Aucoin bronzer in **Tropical Days.**

3 / BECCA Cosmetics Shimmering Skin Perfector in **Moonstone.**

4 / MAC eyeshadow in **Embark** blended out on lash lines.

5 / Anastasia Beverly Hills Waterproof Crème Color Liner in **Jet** on upper lash line and waterline.

6 / Maybelline Great Lash Mascara (false lashes are optional).

7 / Anastasia Beverly Hills Liquid Lipstick in **Dusty Rose.**

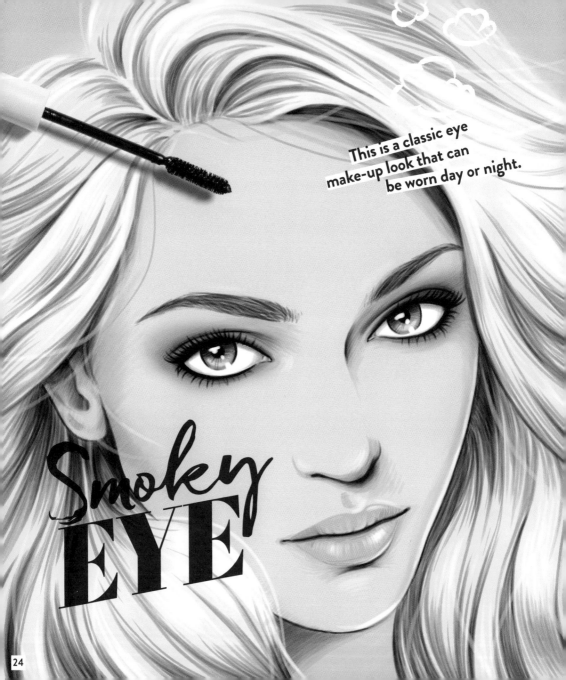

This is a classic eye make-up look that can be worn day or night.

Smoky EYE

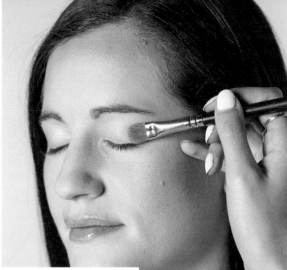

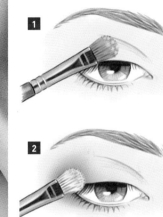

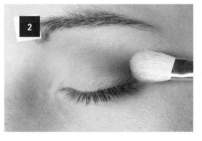

The first thing to do when applying any make-up on your eyes is to prime your eyelids. There are various primers you can use for this but I personally prefer to use foundation and powder. I also apply make-up on the eyelids before anywhere else on the face, in case any product drops down onto the skin beneath the eyes, ruining any foundation/concealer that has already been applied.

1 / After cleansing the face, apply your normal foundation all over your eyelids. This evens out the skin tone, as well as avoiding any creasing that may happen later in the day. Set with a translucent powder.

Start with a **DARKER SHADE** *on the outer corners*

2 / With a flat brush, apply a darker shade in the outer corners of the eye. Using a clean blending brush, gently blend out the eyeshadow to diffuse the colour into your skin. Always start off lightly with little eyeshadow so you can gradually build up the colour to your desired effect. This way you can decide how smoky you want the make-up to be! Keep adding and blending away.

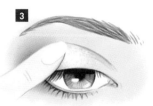

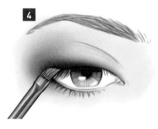

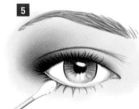

3 / With your (clean) index finger, add a lighter colour to the centre of your eyelid. The warmth from your finger helps products melt into your skin, and works as a perfect blending tool to give a more intense pop of colour.

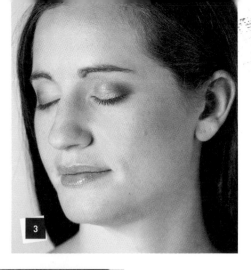

4 / Taking a black or dark brown eyeshadow, draw a line using your upper lash line as a guide. Then gently blend the eyeshadow with a clean blending brush. (If you want a more dramatic look, apply a flick using gel liner for this step.)

5 / Wipe away any excess product that may have fallen down and apply foundation and concealer to the rest of the face (see pages 18–21).

Applying the lighter colour with your finger gives you a more **INTENSE POP** *of colour*

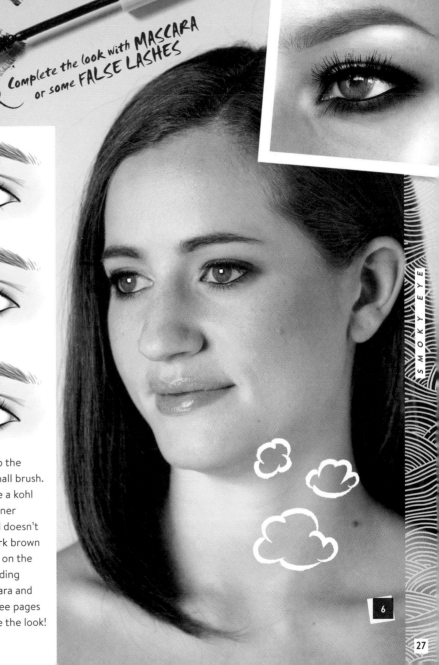

Complete the look with MASCARA or some FALSE LASHES

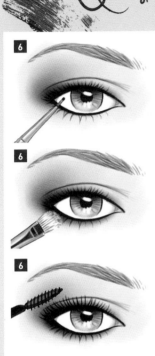

6 / Add a gel liner to the waterline using a small brush. You may want to use a kohl liner, but I find gel liner stays put all day and doesn't smudge. Apply a dark brown or black eyeshadow on the lower lash line, blending out. Then add mascara and some false lashes (see pages 50–53) to complete the look!

Everyday Neutrals

This is a very simple everyday make-up look which will instantly make your eyes appear brighter.

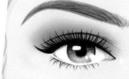

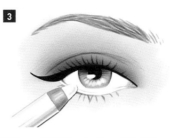

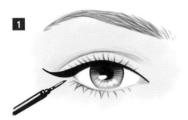

1 / Prep and prime the eyelids (see page 25). Create a wing using Illamasqua Precision Gel Liner (see pages 38–41).

3 / Apply NYX Jumbo Pencil in Milk to the waterline. White eyeliner is great if you are feeling a little tired and want to make your eyes appear wider. This is a must-have product for me and can be used in lots of different ways. It's also great for applying all over the lid before eyeshadow to really help the colour pop.

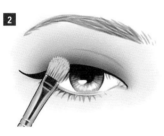

2 / Add a dark brown eyeshadow such as Inglot Matte #329 above the liner and really blend the eyeshadow out. This might diffuse the winged liner that was applied at the beginning, so go back over that again if necessary.

Inglot in **MATTE #329**

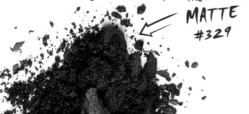

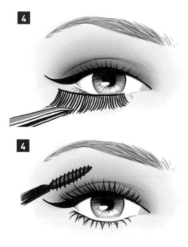

4 / To complete the look, add MAC 33 Lashes with a thin coat of Maybelline Great Lash Mascara in Very Black on the top and bottom lashes (see pages 50–53).

CUT CREASE

A great way to make your eyes appear bigger and brighter!

1 / Prep and prime the eyelids (see page 25). Start off by choosing the transition colour. A transition colour is applied if you're creating a look that has a dark to light colour gradient – the transition colour bridges the gap between the two shades. My favourite to use is Anastasia Beverly Hills eyeshadow in Morocco. Apply this right into the crease with a small blending brush, blending it upwards as you apply.

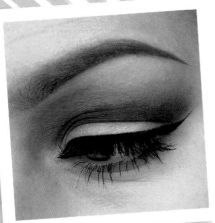

My transition colour, Anastasia Beverley Hills in **MOROCCO**

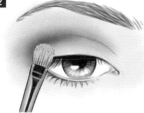

2

2 /
Taking a clean blending brush, sweep on a dark brown eyeshadow such as Mulac Cosmetics in Coffee in the same place as the transition shade, holding the brush at an upward angle. Holding it at this angle means the brush will do a lot of the blending for you. Always start off with less product on the brush and gradually build up the colour in between blending. You can also go back in using the first brush with the transition shade as this will also help to blend and diffuse the darker eyeshadow.

Mulac Cosmetics in COFFEE

3

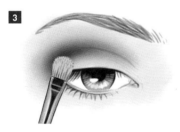

3 /
Add an even darker eyeshadow such as MAC eyeshadow in Carbon to really add depth to the cut crease, again blending it upwards.

MAC in CARBON

4 /
With a flat brush, pack a light shade such as MAC eyeshadow in White Frost all over the eyelid. Be careful not to blend into the cut crease too much as we want to leave a sharp line between these two colours.

MAC in WHITE FROST

4

5 /
Line the eyes with Anastasia Beverly Hills Waterproof Crème Color Liner in Jet.

5

6 /
To complete the look, add Eylure No. 35 Lashes and a coat of mascara (see pages 50–53).

6

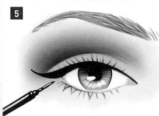

C U T   C R E A S E

Smoky
under eye

This is one of my favourite go-to eye looks if I'm in a rush, as it's so simple to do and I love the finished look.

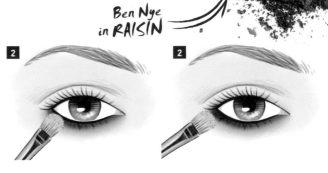

Ben Nye in RAISIN

1 / Prep and prime the eyelids (see page 25). Line the waterline with Anastasia Beverly Hills Waterproof Crème Color Liner in Jet, using a small brush.

2 / Add Ben Nye eyeshadow in Raisin to the lower lash line and blend, gradually diffusing the colour outwards before adding MAC eyeshadow in Sketch. If you want to intensify the look even more, add a black eyeshadow, such as MAC Carbon, to the bottom outer corner of the eye.

3 / To complete the look, curl your lashes and coat generously with Yves Saint Laurent False Lash Effect Mascara.

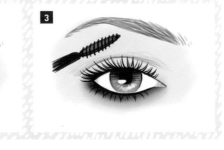

MAC in SKETCH

PURPLE HAZE

**Vibrant violet, lustrous lavender...
lose yourself in a purple haze!**

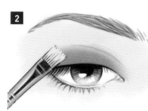

Mulac Cosmetics in **GAME**

1 / Prep and prime the eyelids (see page 25). Apply NYX Jumbo Pencil in Milk all over the eyelid.

2 / With a flat brush, pack on Mulac Cosmetics eyeshadow in Game, blending out at the crease.

3 / With your index finger, pat on Kat Von D Metal Crush eyeshadow in Danzig over the lid, blending away any hard edges.

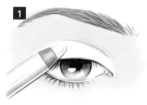

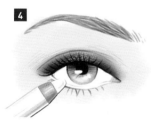

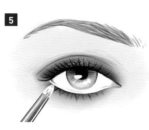

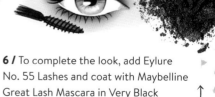

4 / Apply the same NYX Jumbo Pencil in Milk to the waterline.

5 / Taking a small pencil brush, apply Kat Von D Metal Crush eyeshadow in Raw Power under the bottom lash line.

6 / To complete the look, add Eylure No. 55 Lashes and coat with Maybelline Great Lash Mascara in Very Black (see pages 50–53).

Kat Von D Metal Crush in **DANZIG**

Kat Von D Metal Crush in **RAW POWER**

ELECTRIC
BLUE

I know a lot of people may be scared of trying out a blue smoky eye, but I'm a huge fan. It looks great on any skin tone with any eye colour and it's good to try something different. I guarantee you will love it!

Mulac Cosmetics in
TITANIC

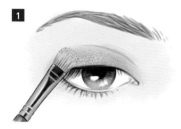

1 / Prep and prime the eyelids (see page 25). Pack Mulac Cosmetics eyeshadow in Titanic all over the lid, blending out at the crease with a small blending brush. Keep adding and blending until you have the desired effect.

2 / Apply MAC eyeshadow in Contrast to the crease and blend out.

Mulac Cosmetics in **CONTRAST**

3 / Create a wing using Barry M Liquid Eyeliner in Turquoise (see pages 38–41).

4 / Line the waterline with Rimmel Kohl Liner in Blue.

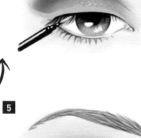

Barry M Liquid Eyeliner in **TURQUOISE**

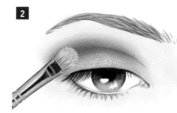

5 / Using the same eyeshadow and brush as in step 1, apply more shadow under the eye and blend out.

6 / To complete the look, add Eylure No. 116 Lashes and a coat of mascara (see pages 50–53).

ELECTRIC BLUE

35

Halo Eye

This make-up looks great teamed with false lashes and will earn you a tonne of compliments!

My transition colour, Anastasia Beverley Hills in MOROCCO →

Ben Nye in RAISIN

1 / Prep and prime the eyelids (see page 25). Use Anastasia Beverley Hills in Morocco as the transition shade, sweeping on with a soft fluffy brush from the outer corner of the eye and blending all along the crease.

2 / Using your finger, pat Ben Nye eyeshadow in Raisin onto the outer third of the eye, diffusing the colour towards the centre of the lid, then do the same on the inner corner of the eye, again diffusing towards the centre, leaving the centre of the lid blank.

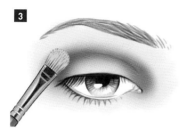

3 / Using the same eyeshadow, connect the colour on the inner and outer part of the eye, creating a halo shape above the centre of the lid in the crease. Use soft strokes with only a small amount of product on the blending brush.

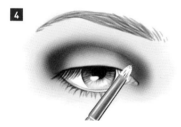

4 / Use a small pencil brush and a darker eyeshadow such as Anastasia Beverly Hills in Beauty Mark to define the halo shape and intensify the colour already applied. This will give your look more depth and dimension. Blend with a clean, soft brush to diffuse any hard edges.

Anastasia Beverly Hills in BEAUTY MARK

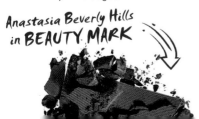

5 / With a flat brush, smooth MAC eyeshadow in White Frost over the centre of the lid, blending the edges into the inner and outer corners.

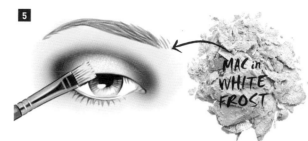

MAC in WHITE FROST

6 / Line the waterline with Anastasia Beverly Hills Waterproof Crème Color Liner in Jet.

7 / Brush Anastasia Beverly Hills eyeshadow in Beauty Mark under the eye and blend outwards.

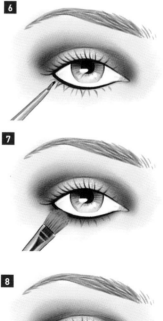

8 / To complete the look, add Eylure No. 035 Lashes and a coat of mascara (see pages 50–53).

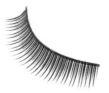

Winged
LINER

Winged liner can be worn alone or used with
many of the eye make-up looks in this book.
It instantly opens up the eyes, so
it's a great skill to perfect!

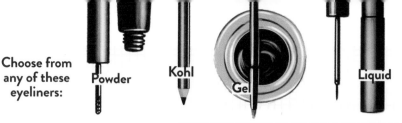

Choose from any of these eyeliners: Powder   Kohl   Gel   Liquid

There are many different ways to apply winged eyeliner and many different products you can use to do so, depending on the look you want to achieve. My favourite eyeliner product is gel liner, with liquid liner on top. The liquid liner on top of the gel makes the black more intense and leaves a crisp, sharp line.

Find the correct angle for the wing by placing your brush in line with the edge of your nostril, pointing up to the tail of your brow.

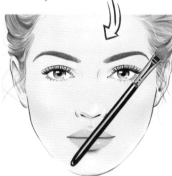

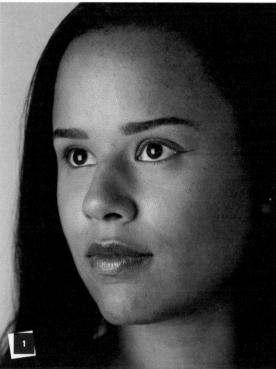

1 / Prep and prime the eyelids (see page 25). Using gel liner and an angled brush, start at the outer corner of your eye, using your lower lash line as a guide, and make one swift stroke. If you draw the line upwards, your eyes will appear wider; if you draw the line outwards, your eyes will appear elongated. Don't be afraid to experiment with the angle and length of the line to find out what suits your eye shape the most and helps you feel most confident!

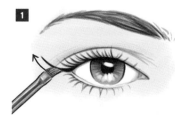

2 / Starting from the tip of the wing you have just created, flip the brush and bring the line back down, creating a triangle shape at the end of your eye. It's most effective to try and do this in a single movement.

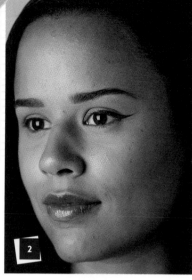

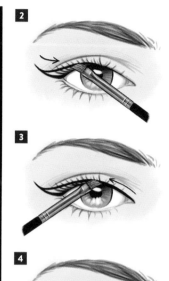

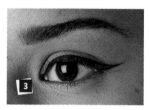

3 / Starting from either the inner corner or the centre of your eyelid (depending on your eye shape and the look you want to achieve) bring the liner towards the triangle, using your lash line as a guide. If you struggle with this part, try drawing smaller lines that you can gradually join together, rather then a single quick sweep with your brush. You can make this line as thick or as thin as you prefer. Starting with a thin line at the inner corner which gradually becomes thicker creates a beautiful cat eye effect.

4 / Fill in the triangle and any other empty space you can see so there are no gaps showing.

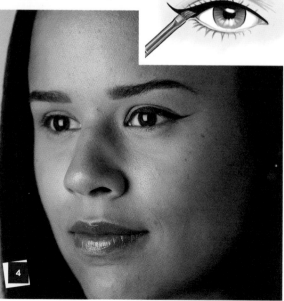

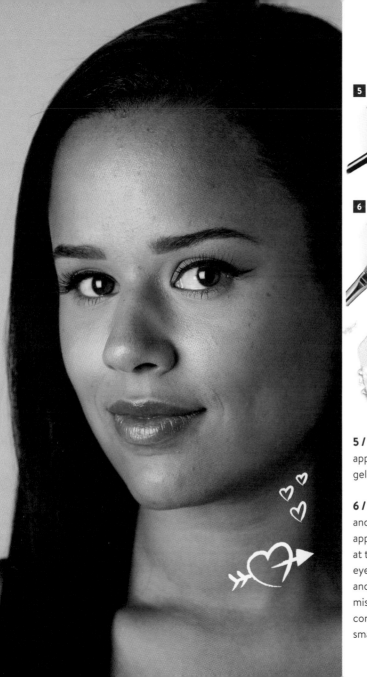

5 / For a more intense look, apply liquid liner over the gel liner.

6 / Take a flat concealer brush and a cream concealer and apply underneath the wing at the outer corner of your eye. This will sharpen the wing and instantly neaten up any mistakes. Blend any visible concealer downwards with small, gentle swipes.

To neaten any mistakes apply a *CREAM CONCEALER* underneath the wing

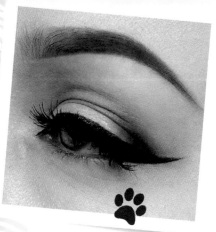

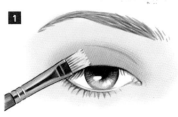

MAC in ALWAYS SUNNY

1 / Prep and prime the eyelids (see page 25). Sweep MAC eyeshadow in Always Sunny over the lid with a flat eyeshadow brush.

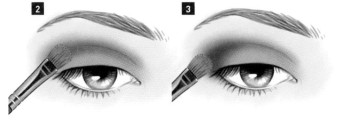

Classic CAT EYE

This is the perfect look to practice that winged liner on! It's the classic cat eye that everyone knows and loves and it's a great way to really elongate the eye.

2 / Brush a small amount of MAC eyeshadow in Charcoal Brown over the crease.

3 / Mix together MAC eyeshadows in Charcoal Brown and Embark, apply to the outer crease and blend.

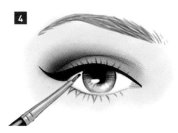

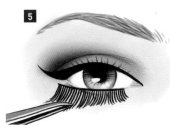

4 / Create a wing using a black liner such as Maybelline Eye Studio Gel Liner (see pages 38–41).

5 / To complete the look, add Eylure No. 155 Lashes and a coat of mascara (see pages 50–53).

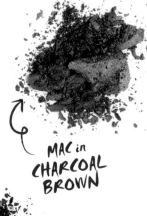

MAC in CHARCOAL BROWN

MAC in EMBARK

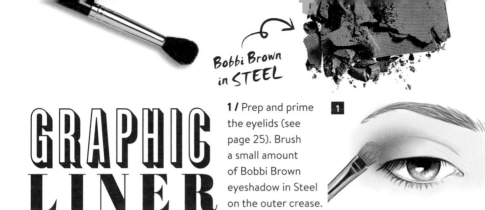

Bobbi Brown in STEEL

GRAPHIC LINER

This is a really fun look to try out and is easier than you think!

1 / Prep and prime the eyelids (see page 25). Brush a small amount of Bobbi Brown eyeshadow in Steel on the outer crease.

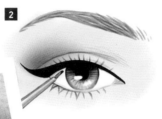

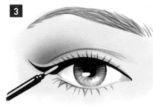

2 / Create a wing using Tarte Clay Pot Waterproof Liner in Black (see pages 38–41).

3 / Draw another wing above using a turquoise liner such as Barry M Liquid Eyeliner, carefully following the line of your black wing. Take your time when applying this – it might help to draw smaller lines and then connect them. If you do make a mistake, use your black liner to touch up any messy areas.

Barry M Liquid Eyeliner in TURQUOISE

4 / To complete the look, add Eylure No. 035 Lashes and a coat of mascara (see pages 50–53).

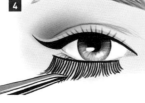

Eyebrow
SHAPING

The shape of your eyebrows can completely change the appearance of your face. Make-up can be used to add depth, fill in any gaps and help your eyebrows appear as symmetrical as possible. (Remember, eyebrows are sisters, not twins!)

There are three different techniques for shaping eyebrows:

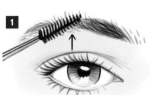

WAXING
Removing hair from the root of the follicle. This gradually starts to reduce hair growth.

THREADING
This works best for sensitive skin. It's an ancient Indian method using cotton thread.

TWEEZING
Effective method for removing unwanted stray hairs.

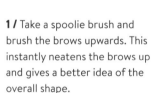

1 / Take a spoolie brush and brush the brows upwards. This instantly neatens the brows up and gives a better idea of the overall shape.

2 / Add a little moisturiser to the brow area and let it soak in. This will help to reduce any pain.

3 / Remove any unwanted stray hairs with tweezers. Ideally, the beginning of the brow should align with the centre of the nostril and the arch should align with the back third of the eye.

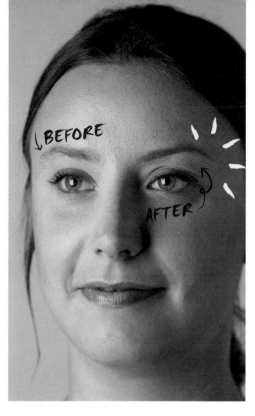

BEFORE

AFTER

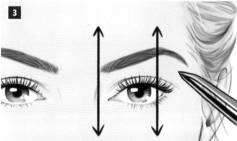

TIP: HOLD A BRUSH against your face to see the ANGLES.

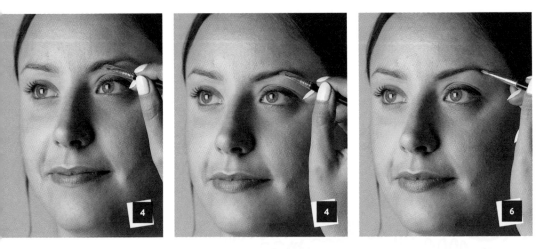

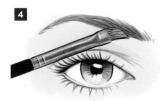

4 / Use a powder in your desired shade – my favourite powders are included in the Anastasia Beverly Hills Brow Pro Palette. Take a thin, angled brush and begin drawing a soft line on the inner edge of the eyebrow.

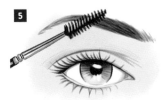

5 / Brush the powder through at an upward angle with the spoolie brush and gradually build up with the product until you have your desired depth. Think of your spoolie brush as you would a blending brush when using eyeshadow. It reduces any harsh edges when adding colour, making the brows appear as natural as possible.

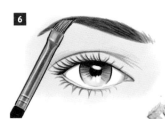

6 / Add a little more powder to the arch of the brow and then bring it down to the tail using one, soft sweep.

Anastasia Beverly Hills Brow Pro Palette

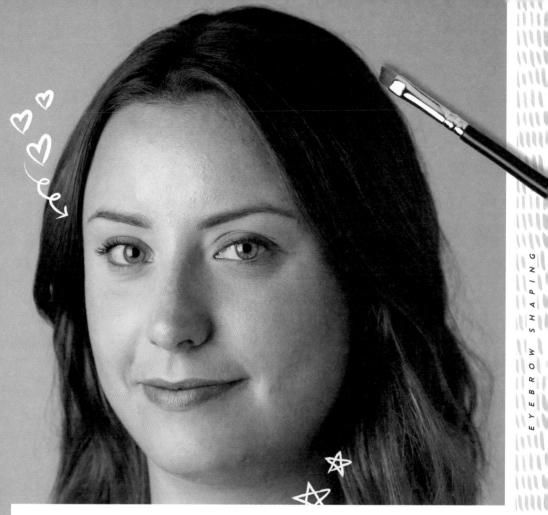

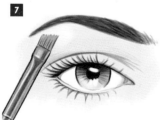

7 / If you want more definition and precision, take a clean angled brush and a cream concealer and apply directly under your brow, making sure it's well blended.

8 / Set with a clear gel.

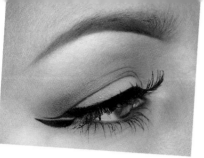

Bobbi Brown in
STEEL

DOUBLE WING

Unique, fun and wearable – I love this look!

Mulac
Cosmetics
in ON

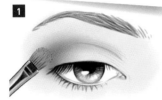

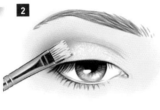

D O U B L E W I N G

1 / Prep and prime the eyelids (see page 25). Apply a small amount of Bobbi Brown eyeshadow in Steel to the crease and blend across the outer corner of the eye. As the wing will be quite dramatic, make sure not to apply too much eyeshadow.

2 / With a flat brush, sweep Mulac Cosmetics eyeshadow in On over the centre of the lid.

3 / Taking Tarte Cosmetics Clay Pot Liner in Black and a thin eyeliner brush, apply a very thin line across the upper lash line, working your way outwards and stopping just before reaching the corner of the outer lash line.

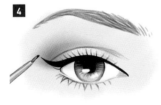

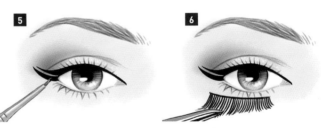

4 / With most winged liner techniques it's best to avoid the crease, but for this look you actually aim to bring the liner into the crease. Draw a wing upwards, making it as thick or thin as you like.

5 / For the bottom wing, use the lower lash line and the first wing as a guide. Follow the same direction as the upper line, leaving a thin gap in between the two. This can be cleaned up with a small angled brush and a cream concealer if necessary.

6 / To complete the look, add Eylure No. 117 Lashes and a coat of mascara (see pages 50–53).

*TIP: The **THINNER** your brush, the easier it will be to apply the liner!*

48

Inverted WING

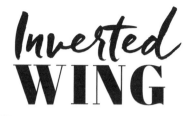

Makeup Geek in PEACH SMOOTHIE

1 / Prep and prime the eyelids (see page 25). Apply a transition eyeshadow such as Makeup Geek in Peach Smoothie along the crease.

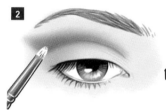

Ben Nye in TAUPE

A smoky mix between a cut crease and winged liner. This is a striking look that suits all eye shapes!

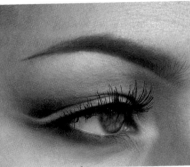

2 / Using a small pencil brush, add a small amount of Ben Nye eyeshadow in Taupe just above the crease and blend out in the same direction as you would a gel winged liner, but a little higher. Make sure the colour diffuses nicely into the skin.

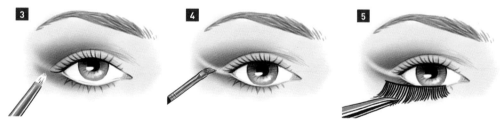

3 / Using the same brush and the Ben Nye Taupe eyeshadow, apply underneath the eye, directly under the pupil, and shade outwards, following the line of the above wing, but leaving a gap between the two.

4 / If the gap starts to look a little messy or the lines of the eyeshadow aren't sharp enough, redefine the gap with a small angled brush and a cream concealer, making sure to leave a soft finish.

5 / To complete the look, add MAC 4 Lashes and a coat of mascara (see pages 50–53).

Applying
FALSE
LASHES

Applying false lashes can sometimes be tricky – here I'll show you how to make it that little bit easier!

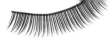

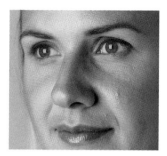

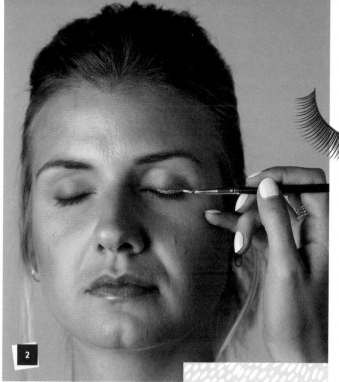

Most packets of false lashes come with glue included, but if not, my favourite glue to use is Duo Striplash Adhesive.

Strip lashes and individual lashes are perfect for finishing off a look. Once you get the hang of applying them, there are so many to choose from, ranging from soft and natural to crazy dramatic.

1 / To start, you need to measure the lashes to fit your eye shape. Place them on your lash line (without glue) and work out where they need to be cut. Cut the outer side of the lashes rather than the inner corners. It's better to cut too little then too much, so take your time with this. Keep going back and measuring until the strip is the same length as your natural lash line.

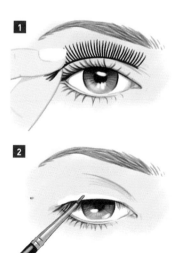

2 / Take a cheap brush (this doesn't have to be a make-up brush – you can buy a thin paintbrush if you wish – the smaller the better) and use this to apply the glue to your upper lash line. If you have drawn on a winged liner, you can use that as a guide, or just follow your upper lash line. It doesn't matter if it's a little messy as the glue turns transparent once dry.

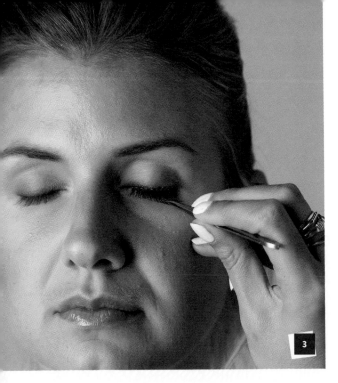

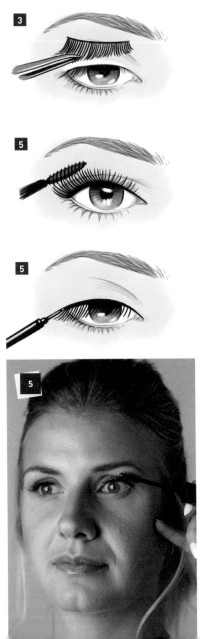

3 / Wait for the glue to get a little tacky and almost transparent, then using your fingers or tweezers (whichever you find easier) place the eyelash strip on top of the glue. Gently hold the lashes in place for 20 seconds.

4 / Make sure there are no areas where the false lashes are digging in uncomfortably. If that does occur, gently peel the lash off and place on your lid again. If you aren't used to wearing lashes it may feel a little strange at first, but after 5 minutes or so you will forget you have them on.

5 / Apply a light coat of mascara to join the natural lashes and the false lashes together. Sometimes the strip of the lashes is made of white thread; if this is the case, go over any white that is showing with a black gel or liquid liner.

TIP: If you wear false lashes regularly, try to get them as close as possible to your **NATURAL LASH LINE**, but avoid putting any glue on your actual lashes. This can cause damage to them in the long term.

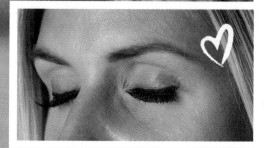

Smoky WING

This look really elongates the eye and leaves an elegant finish.

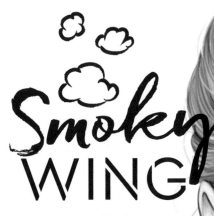

MAC in BLACK TIED

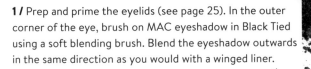

1 / Prep and prime the eyelids (see page 25). In the outer corner of the eye, brush on MAC eyeshadow in Black Tied using a soft blending brush. Blend the eyeshadow outwards in the same direction as you would with a winged liner.

TIP: To create a **SHARP**, straight line, place some scotch tape at the desired angle (usually using your lower lash line as a guide). After packing the product on, gently peel the tape away and it will leave the **CRISPEST** line!

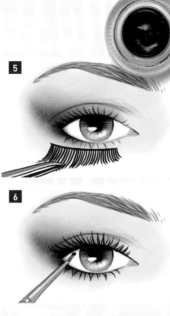

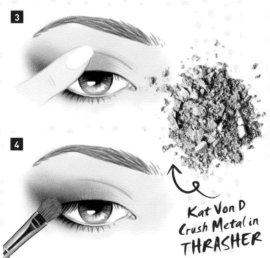

2 / Using the leftover product from the same brush, blend eyeshadow on the lower lash line, right on the outer corner.

Kat Von D
Crush Metal in
THRASHER

3 / Using your index finger, dab a gold eyeshadow such as Kat Von D Crush Metal in Thrasher on the centre of the lid.

4 / Blend the two colours into each other using the same blending brush as before.

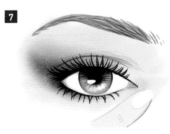

5 / Add Eylure No. 035 Lashes and a coat of mascara (see page 50–53).

6 / Apply Anastasia Beverly Hills Waterproof Crème Color Liner in Jet to the upper lash line.

7 / To complete the look, add a tiny amount of the same gold eyeshadow to the inner corner of the eye with your little finger.

S M O K Y   W I N G

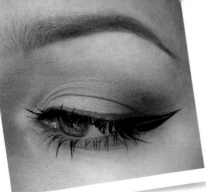

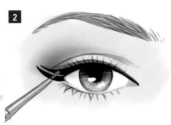

1 / Follow steps 1–4 from the double wing tutorial (see page 48).

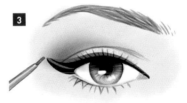

Anastasia Beverly Hills Waterproof Crème Color in EMERALD

GRAPHIC GREEN

This look is similar to the double wing on page 48, but adds a graphic pop of green!

2 / Using a green liner such as Anastasia Beverly Hills Waterproof Crème Color Liner in Emerald and the thinnest eyeliner brush you can find, draw a green line above the black liner, using the upper lash line and the black liner as a guide. Continue the line to the end of the wing.

3 / Fill in the gap between the two black lines using your green liner.

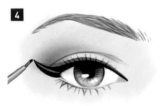

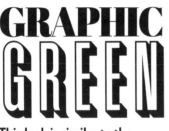

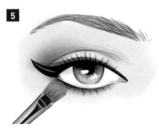

4 / Using your black liner and a thin brush, join the two black wings together to create a triangle shape.

5 / With a soft fluffy brush, apply a green eyeshadow such as Kat Von D Metal Crush in Iggy to the lower lash line.

6 / To complete the look, coat top and bottom lashes with Yves Saint Laurent False Lash Effect Mascara.

Kat Von D Metal Crush in IGGY

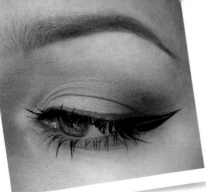

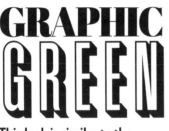

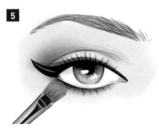

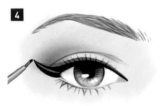

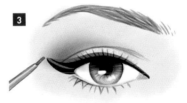

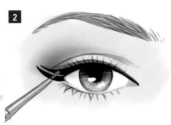

Bold BLACK

Everyone always worries that they'll end up with panda eyes, but take your time, build the colour gradually, and don't forget to blend!

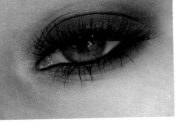

1 / Prep and prime the eyelids (see page 25). Starting with Makeup Geek eyeshadow in Beaches and Cream as the transition colour, apply a generous amount in the crease using a fluffy brush.

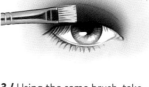

2 / For this look you want to gradually build up the colour. Begin with a dark brown eyeshadow such as Ben Nye in Raisin and pack all over the lid with a flat brush, blending out at the crease.

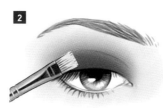

3 / Using the same brush, take a black eyeshadow such as Ben Nye in Black and sweep over the lid. Repeat until the colour is as intense as you like. Keep building up the colour and blending away at the crease.

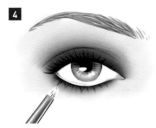

4 / With a small pencil brush and your black eyeshadow, draw along the lower lash line, again building up the colour and blending for a soft look.

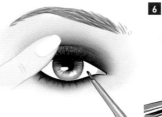

5 / Apply Anastasia Beverly Hills Waterproof Crème Color Liner in Jet to the top and bottom waterlines. For more depth, add Mulac Cosmetics in Off to the centre of the eyelid with your index finger.

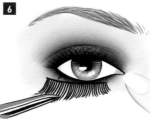

6 / Add Eylure No. 035 Lashes and a coat of mascara (see pages 50–53). With your index finger, dab a small amount of BECCA Shimmering Skin Perfector in Moonstone in the inner corner of the eye to complete the look.

BECCA Shimmering Skin Perfector in **MOONSTONE**

BOLD BLACK

When it comes to highlighting and contouring, I like to customise the look for each individual client. It's best to think of contouring as a way to enhance your face rather than change it.
Try and celebrate your features.
They make you unique!

Highlight
+CONTOUR

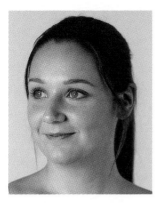

Make-up, in my opinion, is not designed to disguise who you are, but to enhance what you already have. Unique features are what make us beautiful – and more importantly, individuals.

Contouring, as we know it through social media, is all about narrowing the nose, hollowing the cheeks and chiselling cheekbones. Overall, creating illusions.

I don't believe contouring should drastically change the shape of your face. Instead, I like to add subtle definition here and there and then complement with highlighting.

My favourite product to use when contouring is powder bronzer. Whichever product you use, it should be two shades darker than your natural skin tone.

1 / Bronzer is applied after foundation (see pages 18–21). To start off, we need to determine where the bronzer should be applied. Hold a brush up to the side of your face at an angle from the top of your ear down to the corner of your mouth – this is the area you want to shade. Go as near to the ear as you can with a soft, angled brush using gentle, sweeping motions, bringing the colour down and stopping just before the apple of the cheeks. The key to applying bronzer is to blend it out with a clean brush to diffuse the colour, making it appear more natural. Apply with a light hand to gradually build up colour.

TIP:
TAP THE BRUSH a couple of times to remove any excess product before applying.

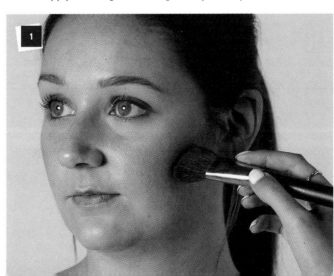

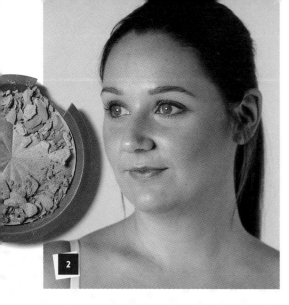

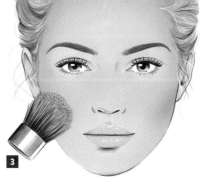

3 / Taking a small of amount of blush, apply gently to the apples of your cheeks, diffusing the two colours together.

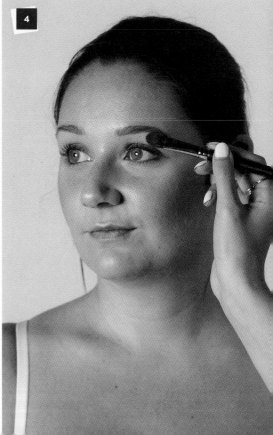

2 / If you would like to make your forehead or jaw appear narrower, lightly sweep on some bronzer at the hairline and/or jawline. Make sure to blend very carefully!

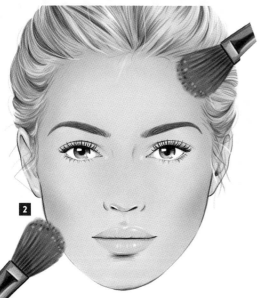

4 / Now you have created shadows on the face, it's time to highlight! Different products work on different skin types so you might have to test out a couple to decide which one works best for you. Our skin can change throughout the year, so you might need to alternate between liquid and powder products! My go-to highlighting product is BECCA Shimmering Skin Perfector. Apply to the cheekbones with a small fan brush, directly above the bronzer. Then, using a smaller brush, dot highlighter on the tip of the nose, Cupid's bow and the inner corner of the eye next to the tear duct.

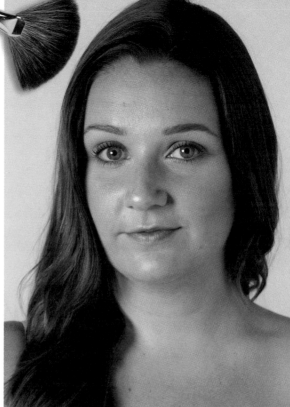

4

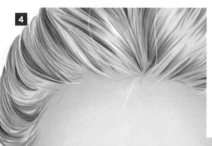

TIP: For a more intense highlight, you can dab on a liquid highlighter (my favourite is **MAC STROBE CREAM**) using your index finger, then apply powder highlight on top as above.

APPLYING *Lipstick*

A pop of lipstick adds glamour to your look in an instant! Learn the steps to achieve that perfect pout.

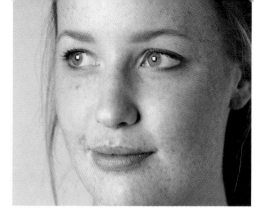

1 / Starting with soft, exfoliated lips, apply a lip primer such as Topshop Lip Primer in Everlast . This will help the lipstick stay on your lips for longer.

The first thing to do when applying lipstick or lip liner is to prep and prime your lips. Covering up chapped lips with lipstick will only accentuate the cracks. Using lip balm has its benefits but regular exfoliation actually removes the dead skin, leaving that soft, plump finish. You can find out how to make my favourite exfoliating lip scrub on page 72, but day-to-day you should gently exfoliate your lips each morning with a toothbrush, pat dry with a towel and add a small amount of lip balm before applying any make-up to your lips.

2 / Lip liner is another big factor in making your lipstick last longer. Try to find a lip liner that roughly matches your choice of lipstick colour. Many brands will have similar colours in both products for this exact reason. Applying lip liner will also stop the lipstick from bleeding (running outside of your lip line).

Apply the lip liner by starting at the Cupid's bow and continue outlining the top lip, following your natural lip line. If you want to make your lips appear fuller, you can apply the liner just above your natural lip line.

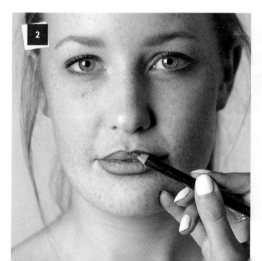

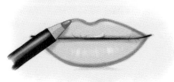

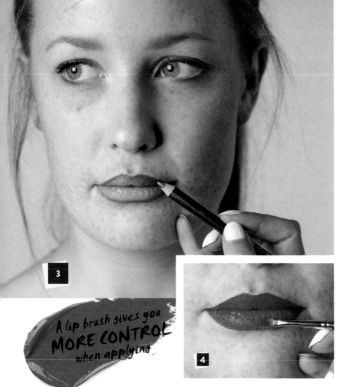

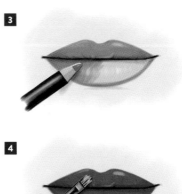

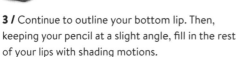

A lip brush gives you
MORE CONTROL
when applying

3 / Continue to outline your bottom lip. Then, keeping your pencil at a slight angle, fill in the rest of your lips with shading motions.

4 / Now it's time for the lipstick! Maintain control by using a lip brush instead of applying the lipstick directly to your lips. Take your time with this and apply as evenly and symmetrically as you can.

5 / If you have made any mistakes or want to sharpen the lines a little, take a concealer brush and apply a small amount of cream concealer to the edges of the lips, making sure the concealer is well blended into the skin. This technique will make the lips really pop.

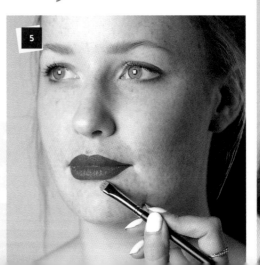

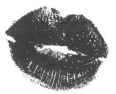

6 / There are several ways to prevent your lipstick from coming off or smudging after application. Place your index finger in your mouth with your lips pressed down and pull it out to stop lipstick getting on your teeth. You can also take a single-ply tissue and place gently over your lips, then take a powder brush with a small amount of loose translucent powder and gently dab over the lips through the tissue. This works as a protective coating for the lipstick. Lastly, you can take a tissue and press your lips down on it for a couple of seconds.

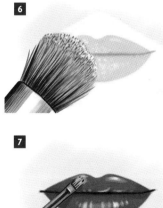

7 / Finally, add some gloss on top if you want a moist, plump effect.

FUN LIPS

Bright Pink

The perfect Barbie lip! This pink from Mulac Cosmetics in Flamingo is so vibrant. As it has a matte formula, it's very long-lasting. You can always add a clear gloss over the top too!

BLUE OMBRE

Mulac Cosmetics in **GUY**

Illamasqua in **DISCIPLE**

An ombre lip is a great way to make your lips appear fuller and it's so easy to create. First, apply Mulac Cosmetics in Guy all over the lips. Then, brush Illamasqua in Disciple on the centre of your bottom lip. To finish off, gently rub your lips together to subtly diffuse the colours into each other.

Mulac Cosmetics in HOPE

This lipstick is quite daring, but the undertones in the colour are actually very flattering and don't leave you looking washed out. But if you don't fancy rocking a green lip to work, Mulac Cosmetics in Hope is perfect for a fancy dress party!

Deep Burgundy

This striking liquid lipstick by Anastasia Beverly Hills in Trust Issues is the perfect colour if you like to rock a bold, darker lip. It complements every skin tone and makes your teeth look pearly white!

Anastasia Beverly Hills in TRUST ISSUES

GREEN

CLASSIC NUDE

Mulac Cosmetics in MOU

My go-to lipstick! You can't go wrong with a classic nude lip. The best nude lipstick can vary from skin tone to skin tone – there are so many varieties out there, so keep trying if you haven't found your perfect one yet. My favourite is Mulac Cosmetics in Mou.

Lip Colours

FOR YOUR SKIN TONE

I'm often asked how to find the most flattering lip colour and my answer generally stays the same...

Wear whatever you feel comfortable wearing, have confidence and know that you can look good in any colour. There are no rules with make-up and it's a great tool to really express yourself and do whatever you want to do.

That said, there are certain colours that can complement your skin tone more then others.

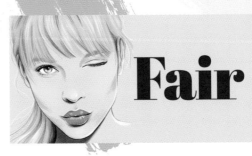

Fair

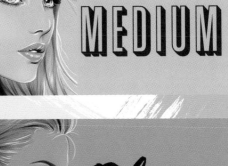

MEDIUM

Olive

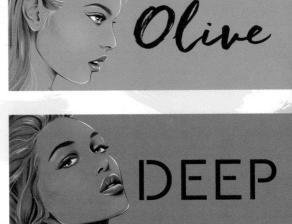

DEEP

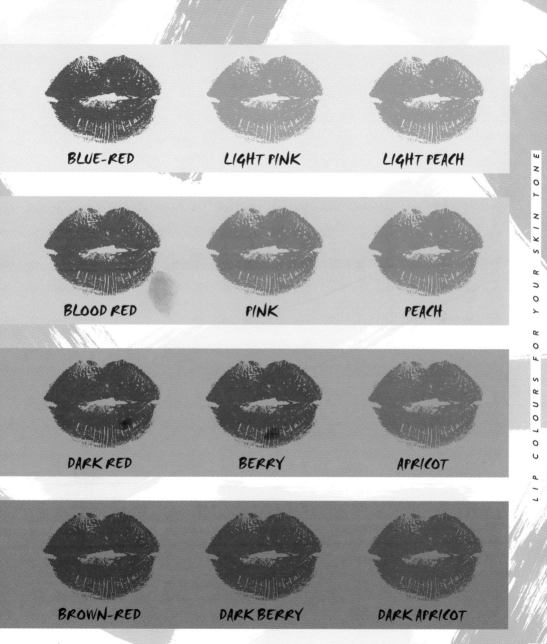

BLUE-RED

LIGHT PINK

LIGHT PEACH

BLOOD RED

PINK

PEACH

DARK RED

BERRY

APRICOT

BROWN-RED

DARK BERRY

DARK APRICOT

Blusher FOR YOUR SKIN TONE

As with lip colours, the blush you choose is entirely up to you, but depending on your skin tone, certain colours might complement your skin more then others.

Always use a light hand when applying blush – the trick is to make it look like the natural colour in your cheeks is coming through, which results in your skin looking awake and rejuvenated and instantly warms your complexion. If there are any harsh lines, you can blend out with your foundation brush to really diffuse the colour into the skin.

TIP: When you're feeling a little **RUN-DOWN** or **TIRED**, dust blush on the apples of your cheeks to give your face a little more **COLOUR**

FAIR

Soft pinks and peaches work best for fair skin tones – not too intense and with just the right amount of subtle colour. My favourite blush for fair skin tones is by MAC in *WELL DRESSED.*

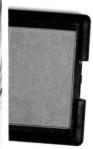

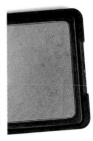

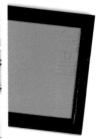

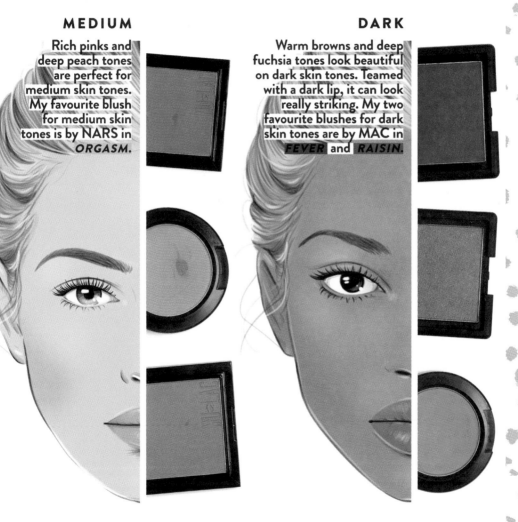

MEDIUM

Rich pinks and deep peach tones are perfect for medium skin tones. My favourite blush for medium skin tones is by NARS in *ORGASM*.

DARK

Warm browns and deep fuchsia tones look beautiful on dark skin tones. Teamed with a dark lip, it can look really striking. My two favourite blushes for dark skin tones are by MAC in *FEVER* and *RAISIN*.

DIY
BEAUTY
PRODUCTS

Whether you need a stocking filler, want to save money, or just like to know exactly what's in the products you're putting onto your face and body, you can't go wrong with these adorable homemade beauty saviours.

DIY:
Lip Balm

Many lip balms include petroleum jelly. However, as lip balm is applied to the mouth and could potentially be ingested, I much prefer to make my own using coconut oil, as it's good for my inside as well as my outside!

YOU WILL NEED:

coconut oil / lipstick in colour of your choice / small container

Instructions: Melt equal amounts of coconut oil and your chosen lipstick in the microwave for 60–90 seconds. Carefully remove from the microwave and mix well with a teaspoon or cocktail stick.

Pour into the container and leave at room temperature until solid. Apply to the lips to moisturise and add a hint of colour!

DIY:
Lip
Scrub

As mentioned on page 63, exfoliating your lips is very important. Exfoliation helps your lips to retain moisture for longer and will prevent them from cracking. It is recommended to use this scrub every week or two, depending on how dry your lips tend to be.

YOU WILL NEED:
olive oil / sugar / honey

Instructions: In a small bowl, mix ½ a teaspoon of olive oil, 2 tablespoons of white sugar and 1 teaspoon of honey. Apply a generous amount of scrub to the lips using your index finger, moving in circular motions all over your top and bottom lip. Do this for a minute or two, then rinse with warm water and pat dry with a towel. This will leave your lips feeling soft and smooth!

Natural
INGREDIENTS

Natural and organic skincare is becoming more popular, which is great! Once you know the best ingredients to use and what's going to work well with your own skin type, you can mix and match to find the best facial scrub for you.

Here are some of the most beneficial products you can try out (not necessarily together):

LAVENDER OIL: Disinfects skin and improves circulation. It also treats respiratory problems.

COCONUT OIL: See page 76 for a whole host of benefits!

SUGAR: A natural source of glycolic acid. This is great for new cell production and helps break down the dead cells that are hanging onto your skin. Best to use on the lips rather than delicate facial skin.

OLIVE OIL: Helps to smooth and nourish the skin. It contains antioxidants that can protect the skin from premature ageing. It also helps prevent free radical damage, which can affect collagen, a protein found in our skin which is vital for skin elasticity. We want our skin to stay firm and supple!

DIY: Coconut Face Mask

I suffer from milia (small bumps under the skin) and so I have a couple of small red scars under my eye area. I started to use this mask and began to see results fairly quickly. Please note, this may not work for all skin types and should not be used too often. Lemon juice can lighten the skin (as well as brightening it) so may cause damage when exposed to the sun. If you wish, you can leave out the lemon juice when making this scrub.

YOU WILL NEED:
lemon / coconut oil / raw honey

Instructions: Take 1 tablespoon of coconut oil and 2 tablespoons of honey and stir until well mixed. Add 1 teaspoon of lemon juice (optional) and stir. Apply the mask to your face, leave for 20 minutes and rinse with warm water. Then pat dry with a towel.

Be careful when using new products on your skin, even when they're natural. PATCH TEST any new skin products on a small area of skin before use and wait at least 24 HOURS before using on the face. Always consult your doctor if you have any skin conditions or problems.

DIY:
Honey
Face Mask

TIP: Scale up the quantities, pour the scrub into **PRETTY JARS** and give to friends as gifts!

There's nothing better then some much-needed pamper time with a nice bubble bath and a face mask. You might not realise that a lot of ingredients in your kitchen can be used for this (the face mask, not the bath)!

Bananas, eggs, milk and even mustard can be great for your skin for a variety of different reasons, but I know none of these sound particularly appealing to apply all over your face.

One of my favourite products to use on the skin is honey. As it's naturally antibacterial, it's great at preventing acne. It is also moisturising and leaves your skin with a beautiful glow. Applying raw honey to a slightly damp face and leaving for about 20–30 minutes will leave your skin feeling smooth and moisturised. You can also try adding some honey to your running bath and soaking your whole body in it.

To enhance that glow even more and really make your skin feel rejuvenated, add some organic orange juice.

THINGS YOU WILL NEED:
honey / orange juice

Instructions: Mix ½ a cup of honey and 3 tablespoons of orange juice. Orange juice is packed full of vitamin C and can help skin look young and replenished. Apply the mask all over your face in circular motions and leave for 30 minutes. Rinse with warm water and then apply your normal moisturiser.

Benefits Of
COCONUT OIL

Coconut oil is quickly becoming one of my favourite products, as it has so many uses! It is great for hair, skin, body... the list goes on! I've included it in lots of my DIY products, and here are a few reasons why it has become so popular and how it could benefit you:

1 Coconut oil is naturally antibacterial and antifungal. In tropical parts of the world, it is used to protect the skin from the sun's harmful rays (SPF 8).

2 It's full of vitamin E, great for repairing skin and preventing premature aging and wrinkling, among many other things!

3 Some psoriasis and eczema sufferers can use it to treat their condition as well as healing any visible damage to the skin. It's also great for anyone battling acne.

4 Coconut oil can be used as a make-up remover, leaving skin feeling soft and rejuvenated.

5 It's great for chapped lips (perfect for the winter months!).

6 Coconut oil is packed full of protein, which keeps skin healthy and fresh.

7 You can even cook with coconut oil – it gives a quick energy boost!

Tackling
SHINE

Beginning the morning with perfectly applied make-up only to glance in the mirror at lunchtime to see a shiny face and half the make-up smudged away has happened to the best of us.

This is because our pores naturally release oils, which keep our skin from drying out. This is great, but sometimes when mixed with make-up it can lead to an oily, shiny face.

But have no fear, there are ways to prevent – or at least reduce – the shine.

MINERAL POWDER *can help absorb excess oil*

Layer slices of **CUCUMBER** *all over*

A GEL LINER *will stay put for a lot longer*

1 / Make sure you wash your face with clean hands. This is to avoid rubbing any oils from your fingers onto your skin.

2 / Use a translucent powder after make-up application. Particularly focus on the T-zone, around the nostrils and chin area.

3 / Research the products that you are using and make sure they are right for your skin type (see pages 10–11).

4 / Try using a mineral powder foundation. These absorb any excess oil your skin may produce.

5 / Don't apply too much of products like moisturiser and primer. Your skin can only absorb a certain amount at once, so if you apply too much it will result in your make-up literally sliding off.

6 / Blot particularly shiny areas with a tissue throughout the day.

7 / If you find your kohl eyeliner smudges throughout the day, try swapping it for a gel liner. These are much more waterproof and stay put for a lot longer.

8 / Exfoliating is a great way to combat oily skin.

9 / If you have an oily skin type, use a good night treatment that is specifically for oily skin – this way your skin will be prepared for the morning.

10 / If all else fails, there are always homemade remedies you can try. Steep a teabag in boiling water, wait for it to cool and lay it on your skin for a few minutes. Or try layering slices of cucumber all over your face!

Holiday
MAKE-UP
BAG

1

2

3

4

5

6

7

We all have our favourite make-up products we wouldn't go anywhere without, but when packing for a holiday it isn't always possible to take everything you want. Less is definitely more on a beach holiday, so I have compiled a list of essential products to take for your week (or two) in the sunshine, including ways to pack bits and bobs without taking up too much space!

1 PRIMER

Laura Mercier Foundation Primer has UVB/UVA protection and is full of vitamins A, C and E, which act as antioxidants that protect the skin from the harmful, aging effects of the environment. It is also extremely lightweight – perfect for hot, sticky climates.

2 FOUNDATION/ BB CREAM

On holiday I tend to wear a BB Cream (BB stands for blemish balm/beauty balm). It works as an all-in-one product to replace moisturiser, foundation and primer. My holiday favourite, YSL Top Secrets BB Cream, has the added bonus of being SPF 25 too.

3 TRANSLUCENT POWDER

Your skin can become very oily on holiday, especially in the evenings with the humid weather, so a long-lasting powder is ideal for your holiday make-up bag. Laura Mercier Translucent Loose Setting Powder is extremely lightweight and leaves skin with a flawless, natural finish, with no caking or creasing.

4 EYESHADOW

MAC has a variety of different sized inserts, which are designed to fit their Pro Palettes. For travelling and on-the-go make-up, I recommend their eyeshadow palette with 15 separate inserts. I have personalised mine with my favourite (mainly neutral) day-to-day eyeshadows. The pallette gives you so much choice and saves loads of space and hassle. Many brands also have the same sized eyeshadows, so you aren't restricted to MAC eyeshadows.

5 BRONZER/ HIGHLIGHTER

Kevyn Aucoin's The Celestial Bronzing Veil gives skin a natural glow and will help you look even more bronzed if you have already caught a little sun. The bronzer uses crystal pigments in silver, bronze and gold so you can also use it to highlight, saving space as there's no need to pack a separate highlighter.

6 WATERPROOF MASCARA

Maybelline Mascara Great Lash Waterproof in Very Black is my holiday must-have! This mascara never clumps and leaves your lashes looking fuller but still natural. Perfect if you want to wear a little make-up while swimming or sunbathing.

7 LIPS

Palmer's Cocoa Butter Moisturising Lip Balm is my holiday essential. I actually use it all year round! It keeps your lips feeling smooth, smells delicious and is the perfect size to keep in your handbag, it has the added benefit of SPF 15 too.

SUNSCREEN

Even if your make-up contains SPF, it's important to use a dedicated sunscreen. My favourite is Garnier Ambre Solaire. Its light formula is moisturising, easy to blend and doesn't leave you looking greasy. No matter what you use, be sure to check the rating for protection from both UVA and UVB rays. Choose a sunscreen with a high SPF, remember to apply 15 minutes before sun exposure and reapply regularly – sunburn isn't a good look for anyone!

HOLIDAY MAKE-UP BAG

FESTIVALL
Inspired

It's great to go a little more dramatic with festival make-up and create something eye-catching. A fun and vibrant style is my go-to festival look. Remember, if you're going for a couple of days, you probably won't want to take a lot of make-up with you, so it might be a good idea to invest in a fun palette that has a range of different colours to choose from.

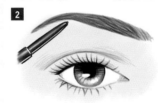

1 / For this look, begin by priming your skin with Laura Mercier Foundation Primer. Depending on how many days into the festival you might be, your skin has most likely seen better days. The primer will help your skin look as fresh and hydrated as possible! Next, prep and prime the eyelids with foundation and translucent powder.

2 / Fill in the eyebrows using Anastasia Beverly Hills Brow Wiz pencil in your colour of choice. Use short strokes to fill in the brow, then blend using the spoolie at the end of the pencil.

3 / Apply a warm brown transition eyeshadow such as Mulac Cosmetics in Toast along the crease with a fluffy brush.

4 / Using the same brush, apply a darker brown eyeshadow such as Mulac Cosmetics in Coffee to the outer corners of the eye, blending away any hard edges.

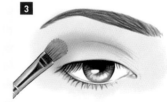

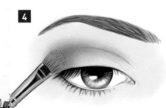

Mulac Cosmetics in TOAST →

Mulac Cosmetics in COFFEE

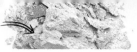

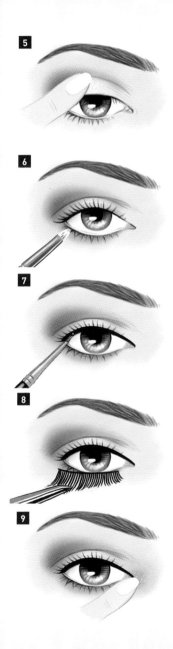

5 / Using your index finger, pat a silver eyeshadow such as Mulac Cosmetics in On all over the centre of the lid.

6 / With a small pencil brush, apply a coral eyeshadow such as Mulac Cosmetics in Miss under the bottom lash line and blend out.

7 / On the upper lash line, apply Anastasia Beverly Hills Waterproof Crème Color Liner in Jet (making sure to create a straight line, not a wing).

8 / Add lashes and a coat of mascara (see pages 50–53). I used Eylure No. 035 Lashes, but go as dramatic as you like! Most brands have a range of fun/fancy dress styles.

9 / Add a splash of bright blue eyeshadow such as Kat Von D Metal Crush in Paranoid to the inner corners of the eye using your index finger. Embrace the messiness!

Kat Von D Metal Crush in PARANOID

10 / For the dots above the eyes, use cream make-up such as Mehron Cream Blend Sticks in Blue and White. Mix 1 part blue make-up to 2 parts white make-up and apply with the smallest brush you can find. Draw four dots above each eye, equally spaced along the eyebrow. Next, outline the right side of each dot with black cream make-up such as Mehron Cream Blend Stick in Black to give a three-dimensional look.

11 / Apply foundation (see pages 18–21).

12 / Finish the look with a pink lipstick such as Black Moon Cosmetics in Libra.

FESTIVAL INSPIRED MAKE-UP

81

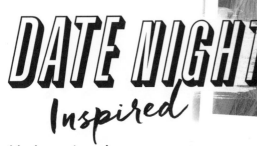

DATE NIGHT
Inspired

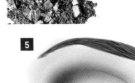

Urban Decay in **NOONER**

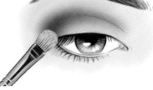

Urban Decay in **DARKSIDE**

It's always nice to have an excuse to dress up! This look is ideal for a nice date or any other special occasion you might have in the diary.

1 / Start by priming the skin with Laura Mercier Foundation Primer.

2 / Apply Yves Saint Laurent Touche Éclat to the eyelids and set with Laura Mercier Translucent Powder.

3 / Fill in the eyebrows using Anastasia Beverly Hills Brow Wiz pencil in your colour of choice. Use short strokes to fill in the brow, then blend using the spoolie at the end of the pencil.

4 / With a blending brush, apply a bronze eyeshadow such as Urban Decay in Nooner in the crease and outer corner of the eye and blend outwards.

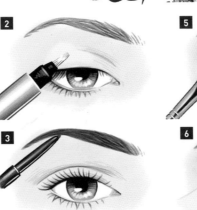

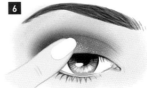

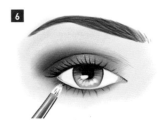

Anastasia Beverly Hills Brow Wiz in **MEDIUM BROWN**

5 / With a clean blending brush, work a dark brown eyeshadow such as Urban Decay in Darkside into the outer corners, blending out and building up gradually until you have the desired effect.

6 / Apply a coral eyeshadow such as Mulac Cosmetics in Miss on the centre of the lid with your index finger. Then take a small pencil brush and apply the same colour directly under the lash line.

7 / Create a wing using a black liquid liner such as Lancôme Artliner in Noir (see pages 38–41).

8 / Before the liquid liner sets completely, use a small angled brush and a black eyeshadow such as MAC in Carbon and brush over the liner, gently blending up to leave a subtle, smoky effect and concentrating on the outer corner of the wing.

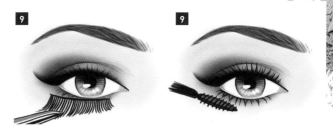

MAC in PEACHES

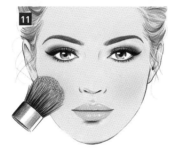
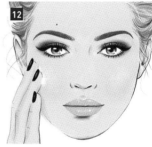

9 / Add Eylure No. 022 Lashes and a coat of Yves Saint Laurent False Lash Effect Mascara (see pages 50–53).

10 / Apply foundation (see pages 18–21).

11 / Sweep MAC Powder Blush in Peaches on the apples of the cheeks, blending well.

12 / Dot BECCA Cosmetics Shimmering Skin Perfector in Opal on your cheekbones.

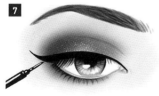

13 / To finish the look, apply Topshop Lip Bullet in Covet to the lips using your index finger, blending out the edges. Dab a tiny amount of Carmex right in the centre of your bottom lip to give the lips a soft, dewy finish.

Topshop Lip Bullet in COVET

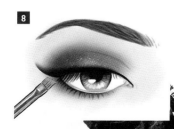

MAC in CARBON

Wedding
Inspired

For wedding make-up, whether you're the bride, bridesmaid or a guest, I believe the focus should be on beautiful skin. There is nothing better than that finished glow for the big day. To give the make-up longevity, the skin will need extra prep. This will help it last throughout the day (and night!).

1 / Start off by applying moisturiser to the skin and leave it to soak in for five minutes.

2 / Spritz MAC Fix+ all over the face, then leave to dry. There is some confusion with this product as some people have been using it as a setting spray, which it isn't! You can apply Fix+ before or after make-up as it helps to create an even surface and refresh the skin. I love to apply it before make-up, then use a setting spray at the end.

3 / Prime the eyelids with foundation and set with a translucent powder.

4 / Using a soft fluffy brush and warm brown eyeshadow such as Mulac Cosmetics in Toast, blend over the eyelid all the way through the crease.

Mulac Cosmetics in TOAST

NOTE: If you are prone to **OILY SKIN**, don't overdo it with products and creams beforehand – this may cause the make-up to gradually slide off as the day goes on.

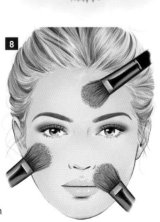
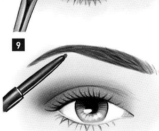
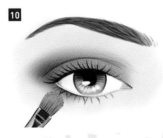

84

5 / Pack a warm dark brown eyeshadow such as Urban Decay in Toasted all over the lid, then add a small amount of a cool dark brown eyeshadow such as Urban Decay in Darkhorse in the outer corners.

6 / Wipe away any-up that may have dropped down underneath the eye using a gentle make-up remover.

7 / Apply foundation – for this look, I chose Yves Saint Laurent Touche Éclat, for a radiant complexion. Next, apply concealer in the necessary areas (see pages 18–21).

8 / With a medium-sized powder brush, dust Laura Mercier Translucent Powder under the eyes, around the nose and mouth and in the centre of the forehead (a small amount goes a long way).

9 / Fill in the eyebrows using Anastasia Beverly Hills Brow Wiz pencil in your colour of choice. Use short strokes to fill in the brow, then blend using the spoolie at the end of the pencil.

10 / Blend a small amount of the cool brown eyeshadow underneath the lash line on the outer corners of the eyes.

11 / Curl your lashes and add a generous amount of Yves Saint Laurent False Lash Effect Mascara.

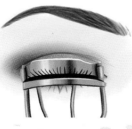

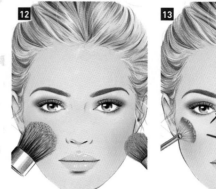

12 / Add a subtle contour using Kevyn Aucoin's The Celestial Bronzing Veil and add a few strokes of Mulac Cosmetics Blush in Bambi on the apples of the cheeks (see pages 58–61).

13 / With a fan brush, highlight the tops of the cheekbones, tip of the nose, Cupid's bow and inner corners of the eye with BECCA Shimmering Skin Perfector in Moonstone.

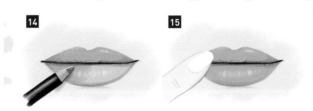

14 / Fill in your lips in with MAC lip liner in Edge to Edge.

15 / To complete the look, add Anastasia Beverly Hills Liquid Lipstick in Pure Hollywood on top, blending out the edges with your index finger (see pages 62–65).

RED CARPET
Inspired

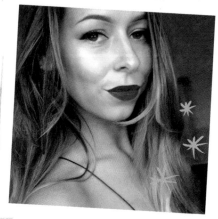

For a sophisticated, glam look I don't think you can go wrong with the classic cat eye teamed with a deep, dark lip.

Yves Saint Laurent Touche Éclat

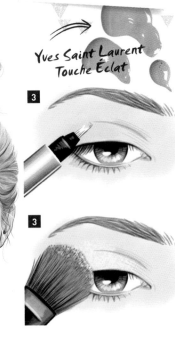

1 / Start off by applying moisturiser to the skin and leave it to soak in for five minutes.

2 / Spritz MAC Fix+ all over the face, then leave to dry.

3 / Apply Yves Saint Laurent Touche Éclat to the eyelids and set with Laura Mercier Translucent Powder.

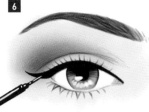

Anastasia Beverly Hills Dipbrow Pomade in **MEDIUM BROWN**

6 / Create a wing using Illamasqua Precision Ink Liner (see pages 38–41). Focus on elongating the eye, keeping the wing fairly straight as opposed to bringing it upwards.

7 / Apply foundation (see pages 18–21).

4 / On the eyebrows, use Anastasia Beverly Hills Dipbrow Pomade in your preferred colour (see pages 44–47).

Anastasia Beverly Hills in **RICH BROWN**

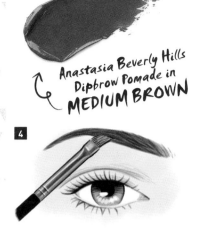

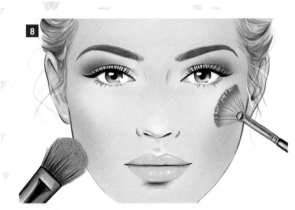

8 / This look suits a more intense bronzer, so apply a generous amount of NARS Laguna Bronzer then highlight with Bobbi Brown Shimmer Brick and a fan brush (see pages 58–61).

5 / Create a subtle cut crease (see pages 30–31) using a deep brown eyeshadow such as Anastasia Beverly Hills in Rich Brown. Leave the centre of the lid clean so the eyeshadow really elongates the eye and draws focus to the wing you are going to make.

9 / To complete the look, apply a deep plum such as Anastasia Beverly Hills Liquid Lipstick in Trust Issues.

DAY to Night

If you're stuck at the office later than you hoped on a Friday evening, or even if you have time to pop home quickly, this quick step-by-step will take you from day to night. It's a great timesaver and will leave you feeling and looking great for your night out.

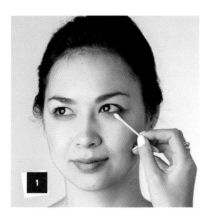

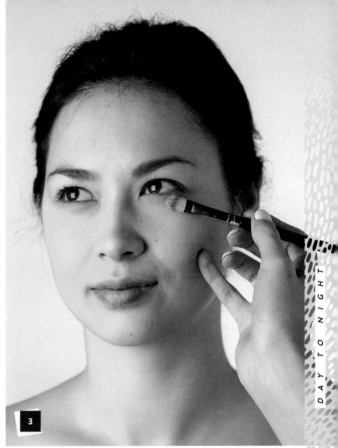

1 / First of all, start by cleaning up any make-up that may have smudged throughout the day, particularly around the eye area. Use a cotton bud with some gentle make-up remover, or even just water.

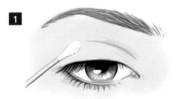

2 / After a long day's work, your skin could probably do with a refresher, so give yourself a generous spritz of MAC Fix+ all over your face. This will make you look and feel more awake.

3 / Apply foundation and/or concealer where necessary, especially under the eyes.

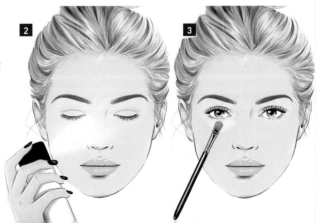

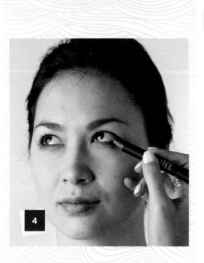

4 / Draw along your upper and lower lash lines with a kohl liner (don't worry if it's messy).

5 / Smudge both lines out with a blending brush.

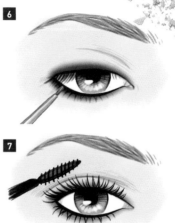

6 / Add some gel liner to the waterline (gel liner is great for a night out as it doesn't budge as easily as kohl does).

7 / Coat top and bottom lashes generously with mascara.

8 / If you feel like you need a little more colour, add a small amount of blush on the apples of your cheeks, and bronzer on your cheekbones.

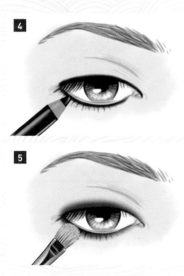

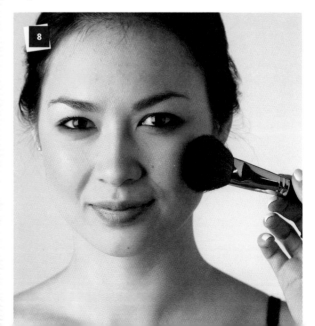

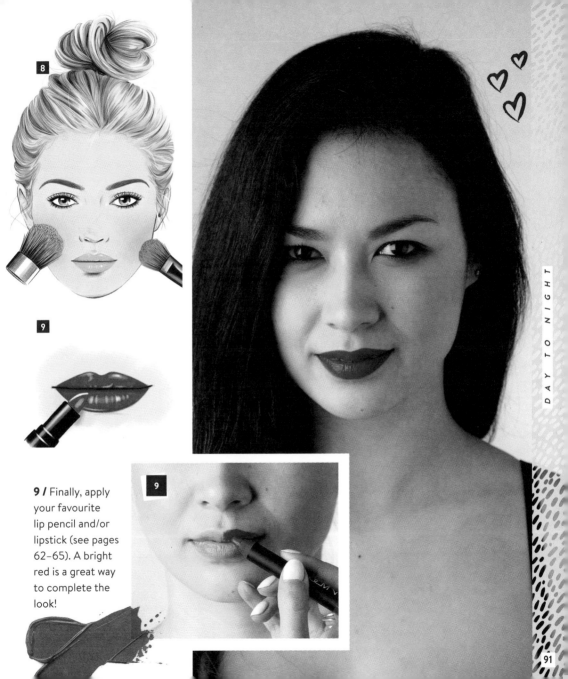

9 / Finally, apply your favourite lip pencil and/or lipstick (see pages 62–65). A bright red is a great way to complete the look!

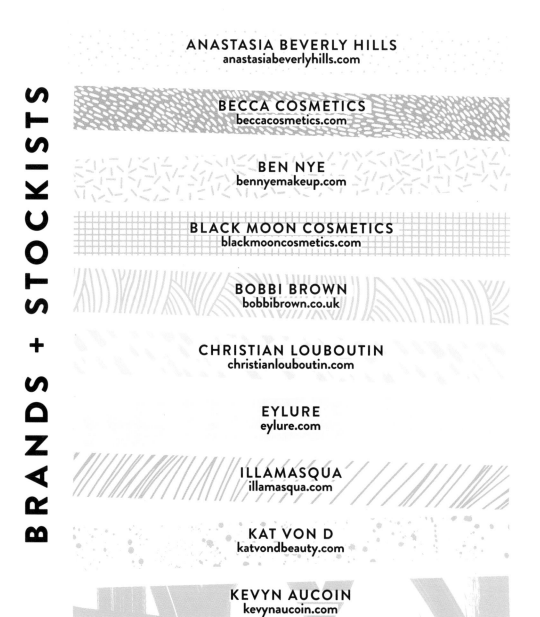

BRANDS + STOCKISTS

ANASTASIA BEVERLY HILLS
anastasiabeverlyhills.com

BECCA COSMETICS
beccacosmetics.com

BEN NYE
bennyemakeup.com

BLACK MOON COSMETICS
blackmooncosmetics.com

BOBBI BROWN
bobbibrown.co.uk

CHRISTIAN LOUBOUTIN
christianlouboutin.com

EYLURE
eylure.com

ILLAMASQUA
illamasqua.com

KAT VON D
katvondbeauty.com

KEVYN AUCOIN
kevynaucoin.com

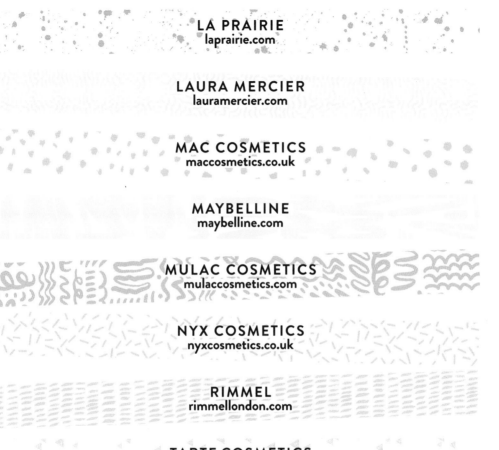

LA PRAIRIE
laprairie.com

LAURA MERCIER
lauramercier.com

MAC COSMETICS
maccosmetics.co.uk

MAYBELLINE
maybelline.com

MULAC COSMETICS
mulaccosmetics.com

NYX COSMETICS
nyxcosmetics.co.uk

RIMMEL
rimmellondon.com

TARTE COSMETICS
tartecosmetics.com

URBAN DECAY
urbandecay.com

YSL
ysl.com

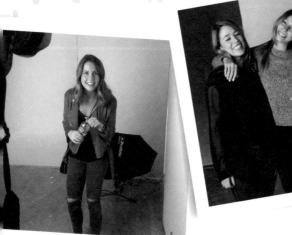

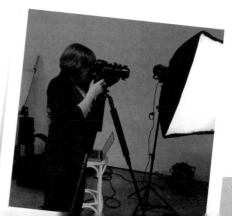

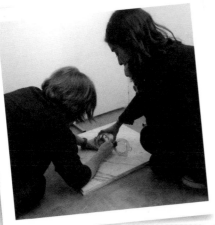

THANK YOU!

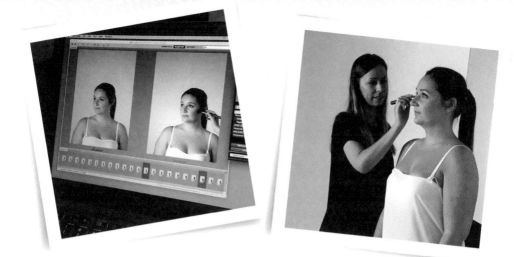

A huge thank you to my friends Hay, Ali, Hails, Lilly, Fee, Jauss, Chanelle and Anastasia. I couldn't have done this without your beautiful faces.

Kate, Kajal, Jacqui, Hannah and Julia, thank you for believing in me, for making this possible and bringing it all to life.

And Alex, thank you for your continuous support and encouragement and for giving me the most cherished advice I have ever received... 'Just blag it.'

Laura Jenkinson

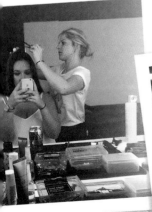

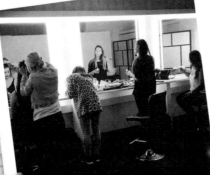

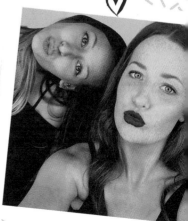

Made Up by Laura Jenkinson

First published in 2016 by Hardie Grant Books

Hardie Grant Books (UK)
52-54 Southwark Street
London SE1 1UN
hardiegrant.co.uk

Hardie Grant Books (Australia)
Ground Floor, Building 1
658 Church Street
Melbourne, VIC 3121
hardiegrant.com.au

British Library Cataloguing-in-Publication Data. A catalogue record
for this book is available from the British Library.

ISBN: 978-1-78488-034-7

Publisher: Kate Pollard
Senior Editor: Kajal Mistry
Editorial Assistant: Hannah Roberts
Photography: Jacqui Melville
Art Direction and Illustrations: Julia Murray
iStock images on pages: 8, 9, 35, 37, 51, 86,
Shutterstock images on pages: 8, 14, 20, 23, 26, 30, 31, 33, 35, 36, 37,
43, 48, 55, 56, 64, 66, 67, 77, 80, 81, 82, 83, 84, 85, 87, 91
Colour Reproduction by p2d

Printed and bound in China by 1010

10 9 8 7 6 5 4 3 2 1